GASTROPARESIS DIET RECIPES COOKBOOK

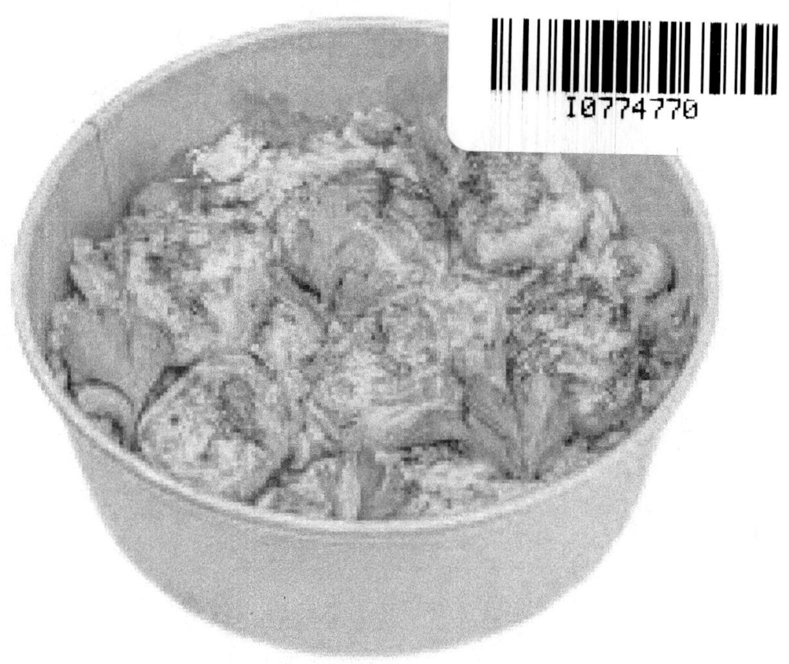

30+ Nutritious, Healthy and Flavorful Meal Plan for a

Stomach Relief

Isabelle Hartley

i

OTHER BOOKS BY THIS AUTHOR

1. RECIPES FOR LOW BLOOD CHOLESTEROL
2. ATKINS DIET RECIPES COOKBOOK
3. CARDIAC DISEASE DIET COOKBOOK
4. CELIAC DISEASE RECIPES COOKBOOK
5. JUICING RECIPES FOR CANCER
6. CIRRHOSIS DIET RECIPES COOKBOOK
7. ADRENAL-STRESS RELIEF COOKBOOK
8. DIABETES DIET RECIPES FOR BEGINNER
9. POSTRATE CANCER DIET RECIPES
10. HIGH CALORIES DIET COOKBOOK

TABLE OF CONTENTS

INTRODUCTION

This thorough guide to embracing a purposeful and delicious approach to fueling your body while navigating the obstacles of gastroparesis is the Gastroparesis Diet Cookbook.

Gastroparesis, a condition affecting the normal movement of muscles in your stomach, can present unique dietary challenges. This cookbook is not just a collection of recipes; it's a roadmap to redefining your relationship with food. Through careful consideration of ingredients and meal plans, we aim to empower you to take control of your nutrition, making choices that can alleviate symptoms and enhance your overall well-being.

The introduction chapters delve into understanding Gastroparesis—its causes, symptoms, and the crucial role of nutrition in managing this condition. We explore the science behind the Gastroparesis diet, providing you with insights into how specific foods and dietary patterns can positively impact your digestive health.

Navigating a Gastroparesis-friendly diet doesn't mean sacrificing flavor or variety. Our cookbook is filled with diverse, mouthwatering recipes crafted to meet the nutritional needs of individuals with Gastroparesis. From nourishing smoothies to easily digestible soups and innovative main courses, each recipe is thoughtfully designed to prioritize both taste and nutritional value.

In addition to recipes, this cookbook offers practical tips for meal planning, grocery shopping, and dining out with Gastroparesis. We believe that knowledge is key to empowerment, and by understanding the principles of a Gastroparesis-friendly diet, you'll be equipped to make informed choices that support your health goals.

Join us on this culinary journey as we embrace the ability of food to treat or reverse gastroparesis. With the help of this cookbook, you can prepare tasty, healthful meals that meet your specific dietary requirements and promote a revitalized feeling of energy and wellbeing.

Justina Story

Meet Justina, a remarkable individual whose journey with Gastroparesis underwent a transformative shift with the help of the principles outlined in this cookbook. Justina's story is a testament to the potential for positive change through mindful nutrition and a Gastroparesis-friendly diet.

Struggling with debilitating symptoms, Justina found herself searching for a solution that extended beyond conventional treatments. Upon discovering this Gastroparesis Diet Cookbook, she embraced its holistic approach to nutrition as a complementary strategy for managing her condition.

Justina saw a noticeable improvement in her symptoms as she followed the cookbook's recipes and accepted its dietary ideas. The carefully curated meals not only eased the strain on her digestive system but also reignited her love for food. Justina's success is not just about symptom management; it's about reclaiming a sense of normalcy and joy in her daily life.

Through sharing Justina's journey, this cookbook aims to inspire and motivate others facing the challenges of Gastroparesis. Her experience serves as a beacon of hope, demonstrating that with dedication to a Gastroparesis-friendly diet, individuals can achieve positive outcomes and regain control over their health.

Justina's success story is a reminder that every small dietary choice can contribute to significant improvements in one's well-being. Use Justina's story as inspiration and motivation as you set out on your own Gastroparesis journey. Together, let's explore the transformative potential of nutrition and embrace the possibility of a healthier, more vibrant future.

CHAPTER 1: GASTROPARESIS

Gastroparesis is a gastrointestinal disorder characterized by delayed emptying of the stomach contents into the small intestine, leading to impaired digestion. This condition can significantly impact an individual's quality of life, causing a range of symptoms and requiring careful management. Let's explore the types, causes, and symptoms of Gastroparesis in detail.

Types of Gastroparesis:

1. Idiopathic Gastroparesis: This is the most common type, where the cause of delayed stomach emptying is unknown.

Idiopathic Gastroparesis often presents with symptoms without an apparent underlying medical condition.

2. Diabetic Gastroparesis:

- Linked to diabetes mellitus, this type occurs due to damage to the vagus nerve, which controls stomach muscles.

- Poorly controlled blood sugar levels can contribute to nerve damage, leading to delayed gastric emptying.

3. Post-Surgical Gastroparesis:

- Sometimes, surgery on the stomach or vagus nerve can result in Gastroparesis.
- Surgical procedures may inadvertently damage the nerves or disrupt the normal functioning of the stomach.

4. Viral Gastroparesis:

- Caused by a viral infection affecting the stomach nerves.
- Certain viruses can lead to inflammation of the stomach nerves, contributing to delayed emptying.

Causes of Gastroparesis:

1. Nerve Damage:

- Vagus Nerve Dysfunction: The vagus nerve controls stomach muscles; damage to this nerve disrupts normal digestion.

- Post-Surgical Complications: Surgical procedures on the stomach or nearby organs can lead to nerve damage.

2. Muscle Dysfunction:

- Smooth Muscle Disorders: Conditions affecting the muscles of the stomach can impede proper contractions for digestion.
- Medication-Induced Dysfunction: Certain medications can interfere with stomach muscle function.

3. Hormonal Changes: Diabetes Mellitus: High and fluctuating blood sugar levels in diabetes can damage nerves, including those regulating digestion.

4. Autoimmune Factors: Inflammatory Disorders: Conditions such as lupus or scleroderma can lead to inflammation affecting the digestive system.

5. Viral Infections: Herpes Zoster Virus: This virus, commonly causing shingles, can affect stomach nerves.

Symptoms of Gastroparesis:

1. Nausea and Vomiting: Recurrent feelings of nausea, and vomiting may occur, especially after meals.

2. Abdominal Pain: Persistent or intermittent pain in the abdomen, often described as a dull ache.

3. Bloating and Fullness: Sensation of fullness after eating small amounts of food, accompanied by abdominal bloating.

4. Heartburn or GERD: Gastroparesis can lead to gastroesophageal reflux disease (GERD) symptoms, such as heartburn.

5. Fluctuations in Blood Sugar Levels: Diabetic Gastroparesis can cause erratic blood sugar levels due to delayed digestion.

6. Malnutrition and Weight Loss: In severe cases, malnutrition and unintentional weight loss may occur due to inadequate nutrient absorption.

7. Erratic Blood Sugar Levels: Diabetic Gastroparesis can cause erratic blood sugar levels due to delayed digestion.

8. Changes in Appetite: Some individuals may experience a loss of appetite or aversion to certain foods.

9. Fatigue: The effort the body exerts to digest food inefficiently can lead to fatigue.

Diagnosis and Treatment:

1. Diagnosis: Clinical History and Physical Exam: A healthcare provider will review symptoms and medical history.

- Imaging Studies: Tests like gastric emptying scintigraphy can confirm delayed stomach emptying.
- Electro-gastrography (EGG): Measures electrical activity in the stomach.

2. Treatment:

- Dietary Modifications: Adjusting the diet to include easily digestible foods and smaller, more frequent meals.
- Medications: Prokinetic drugs to stimulate stomach muscle contractions and antiemetics to control nausea.

- Nutritional Support: In severe cases, nutrition may be supported through tube feeding or, in rare instances, intravenous feeding.
- Surgical Intervention: In extreme cases, surgery may be considered to either remove an obstruction or implant a gastric stimulator.

Gastroparesis, with its varied types and causes, presents a complex challenge for those affected. Recognizing the symptoms and seeking timely diagnosis and treatment are crucial for managing the condition effectively. While there is no cure for Gastroparesis, a multidisciplinary approach involving dietary adjustments, medications, and, in some cases, surgery, can significantly improve symptoms and enhance the quality of life for individuals living with this condition. Understanding the interplay of factors contributing to Gastroparesis empowers both patients and healthcare providers to tailor interventions that address the specific needs of each individual, fostering a more targeted and effective approach to managing this challenging gastrointestinal disorder.

CHAPTER 2: DIETS

FOODS

A Gastroparesis diet plays a crucial role in managing symptoms and improving overall well-being for individuals with this gastrointestinal disorder. Since delayed stomach emptying is a hallmark of Gastroparesis, dietary choices focus on foods that are easier to digest, minimizing stress on the digestive system. Here's a breakdown of foods to include and avoid in a Gastroparesis diet.

Foods to Include:

1. Low-Fiber Foods: Opt for easily digestible, low-fiber options to reduce the workload on the digestive system. Examples: Refined grains like white rice, white bread, and low-fiber cereals.

2. Well-Cooked Vegetables:

   - Cooking vegetables until they are soft can make them easier to digest.

   - Examples: Carrots, zucchini, and spinach (well-cooked).

3. Lean Proteins:

- Choose lean sources of protein to provide essential nutrients without excess fat.

- Examples: Skinless poultry, fish, tofu, and well-cooked eggs.

4. Low-Fat Dairy:

- Opt for low-fat or fat-free dairy to reduce the intake of hard-to-digest fats.

- Examples: Skim milk, yogurt, and low-fat cheeses

5. Soft Fruits:

- Choose fruits that are ripe and soft, making them easier to chew and digest.

- Examples: Bananas, melons, and peaches (canned or fresh).

6. Soups and Broths:

- Liquid-based meals, such as soups and broths, can be gentler on the digestive system.

- Examples: Clear vegetable or chicken broth, pureed soups.

7. Nut Butters:

- Nut butters provide a good source of protein and healthy fats in a more easily digestible form.

- Examples: Almond butter, peanut butter (smooth).

8. Cooked Grains:

- Well-cooked grains offer a source of carbohydrates without excessive fiber.

- Examples: Quinoa, couscous, and white rice.

9. Herbs and Spices:

- Mild herbs and spices can add flavor without causing irritation.

- Examples: Basil, mint, and a touch of ginger.

Foods to Avoid:

1. High-Fiber Foods:

- High-fiber foods can be harder to digest and may exacerbate symptoms.

- Examples: Whole grains, raw vegetables, and legumes.

2. Fatty Foods:

   -   High-fat foods can delay stomach emptying and contribute to discomfort.

   - Examples: Fried foods, fatty cuts of meat, and full-fat dairy

3. Gas-Producing Foods:

   -   Foods that produce gas can lead to bloating and discomfort.

   -   Examples: Carbonated beverages, beans, and cruciferous vegetables.

4. Tough Meats:

   - Tough meats can be challenging to digest, increasing the workload on the stomach.

   - Examples: Steak, pork chops, and other tough cuts.

5. Citrus Fruits:

   - Citrus fruits can be acidic and may cause irritation.

   - Examples: Oranges, grapefruits, and lemons.

6. Caffeine and Alcohol:

- Both caffeine and alcohol can contribute to irritation and slow digestion.

- Examples: Coffee, tea, and alcoholic beverages.

7. Large Meals:

- Consuming large meals can overwhelm the stomach, leading to discomfort.

- Recommendation: Opt for smaller, more frequent meals.

8. Spicy Foods:

- Spicy foods may cause irritation and exacerbate symptoms.

- Examples: Hot peppers, chili, and heavily spiced dishes.

Crafting a Gastroparesis-friendly diet involves thoughtful consideration of food choices to alleviate symptoms and promote better digestion. While individual responses to foods may vary, the overarching principles include prioritizing easily digestible, low-fiber options and avoiding those that may cause irritation or delay stomach emptying. Working closely with healthcare professionals and dietitians can help tailor a Gastroparesis diet to individual needs, fostering a balanced and nutritious approach that supports overall well-being for those navigating the challenges of this gastrointestinal condition.

BENEFITS

Adhering to a Gastroparesis diet can yield a range of core benefits, significantly improving the quality of life for individuals grappling with this gastrointestinal disorder. Through modifying food choices to address the difficulties caused by delayed stomach emptying, people can alleviate symptoms and promote general health. The main advantages of sticking to a gastroparesis diet are as follows:

1. Symptom Management: A Gastroparesis diet is strategically crafted to ease the burden on the digestive system, reducing symptoms such as nausea, vomiting, abdominal pain, and bloating. By choosing easily digestible foods, individuals can better manage the challenges associated with delayed stomach emptying.

2. Improved Nutrient Absorption: Gastroparesis can lead to malnutrition due to inadequate absorption of nutrients. A

well-designed diet ensures that individuals receive essential vitamins and minerals from easily digestible foods, supporting overall health and preventing nutritional deficiencies.

3. Stabilized Blood Sugar Levels (for Diabetic Gastroparesis): For individuals with diabetic Gastroparesis, managing blood sugar levels is crucial. A Gastroparesis diet, focused on low-fiber and easily digestible foods, can contribute to more stable blood sugar levels, reducing the risk of erratic glucose fluctuations.

4. Enhanced Digestive Comfort: By avoiding foods that can exacerbate Gastroparesis symptoms, such as high-fiber or fatty foods, individuals can experience enhanced digestive comfort. This can lead to a reduction in abdominal pain, discomfort, and a general improvement in overall well-being.

5. Prevention of Complications: Gastroparesis, if left unmanaged, can lead to complications such as bacterial overgrowth, bezoars (solid masses of undigested food), and worsening of symptoms. A Gastroparesis diet helps mitigate the risk of these complications by promoting

optimal digestion and minimizing stress on the digestive system.

6. Weight Management: Gastroparesis can contribute to unintended weight loss due to reduced food intake and inefficient digestion. A carefully planned diet ensures that individuals receive sufficient calories and nutrients, supporting weight maintenance and preventing excessive weight loss.

7. Increased Energy Levels: Consuming easily digestible foods in smaller, more frequent meals can help distribute energy intake throughout the day. This approach prevents the energy drain associated with digesting large, heavy meals, leading to increased energy levels and reduced fatigue.

8. Enhanced Quality of Life: By alleviating symptoms, supporting nutritional needs, and promoting overall digestive comfort, a Gastroparesis diet contributes to an enhanced quality of life. Individuals are better equipped to engage in daily activities without the hindrance of persistent gastrointestinal challenges.

9. Empowerment Through Dietary Choices: Following a Gastroparesis diet empowers individuals to take an active role in managing their health. By understanding which foods support optimal digestion and which may exacerbate symptoms, individuals gain a sense of control over their dietary choices, contributing to a more positive outlook on their Gastroparesis journey.

10. Support for Medication Effectiveness: For individuals using medications to manage Gastroparesis symptoms, a complementary Gastroparesis diet can enhance the effectiveness of these treatments. Medications work more efficiently when the digestive system is not overwhelmed by challenging-to-digest foods.

In conclusion, a Gastroparesis diet is a valuable tool in the comprehensive management of this gastrointestinal condition. The core benefits extend beyond symptom relief to encompass improved nutrient absorption, stabilized blood sugar levels, and an overall enhancement of the individual's well-being. By embracing a Gastroparesis-friendly diet, individuals can navigate their daily lives with greater comfort, confidence, and a proactive approach to their health.

How to Follow This Gastroparesis Diet

To reduce symptoms and improve digestion, a gastroparesis diet requires careful planning and a deliberate approach to food selection. The goal is to ease the workload on the digestive system, considering the delayed stomach emptying characteristic of Gastroparesis. Here's a comprehensive guide on how to follow a Gastroparesis diet:

1. Consultation with Healthcare Professionals:

: It is crucial to speak with medical experts, such as a gastroenterologist and a qualified dietitian, before starting a gastroparesis diet. They can provide personalized guidance based on individual health needs and medical history.

2. Identify Trigger Foods: Keep a food journal to identify specific foods that trigger or worsen Gastroparesis symptoms. This can help tailor the diet to individual sensitivities.

3. Meal Frequency and Portion Control: Instead of three large meals, opt for five to six smaller, well-balanced meals throughout the day. Smaller portions are easier to digest and reduce the strain on the digestive system.

4. Choose Easily Digestible Foods: Select foods that are easy to digest, such as well-cooked vegetables, lean proteins, and low-fiber options. These choices minimize the time and effort required for digestion.

5. Avoid High-Fat and High-Fiber Foods: Steer clear of high-fat and high-fiber foods, as they can delay stomach emptying. Opt for low-fat alternatives and choose grains, fruits, and vegetables with lower fiber content.

6. Opt for Well-Cooked Vegetables: Vegetables should be well-cooked to enhance digestibility. Steaming or boiling vegetables until they are soft can make them easier on the stomach.

7. Incorporate Lean Proteins: Choose lean protein sources, such as skinless poultry, fish, tofu, and well-cooked eggs. These provide essential nutrients without excessive fat, promoting easier digestion.

8. Include Soft Fruits: Select soft and ripe fruits, such as bananas, melons, and peaches (canned or fresh). Avoid acidic fruits that may irritate the digestive system.

9. Consider Nut Butters: Nut butters like almond or peanut butter (smooth) can be a good source of protein and healthy fats in a more easily digestible form.

10. Experiment with Soups and Broths: Liquid-based meals, like clear vegetable or chicken broth and pureed soups, can be gentler on the digestive system, providing nourishment without excessive effort.

11. Monitor Fluid Intake: Stay adequately hydrated, but avoid consuming large amounts of liquids with meals, as this can contribute to feelings of fullness and discomfort.

12. Be Mindful of Medications: Consider the timing of medications in relation to meals. Some medications may be more effective when taken with or after food, while others may be more suitable on an empty stomach.

13. Limit Caffeine and Alcohol: Both caffeine and alcohol can irritate the digestive system. Limit their consumption

and consider alternatives like herbal teas or non-caffeinated beverages.

14. Listen to Your Body: Pay attention to how your body responds to different foods. If certain foods consistently cause discomfort, consider removing or minimizing them in your diet.

15. Regular Follow-Up with Healthcare Team: Schedule regular follow-up appointments with your healthcare team to discuss your progress, address any challenges, and make necessary adjustments to your Gastroparesis diet plan.

Adhering to a Gastroparesis diet involves a combination of informed food choices, portion control, and regular monitoring of individual responses. The key is to prioritize easily digestible foods, avoid triggers, and maintain a balanced approach to nutrition. By working closely with healthcare professionals and making personalized adjustments based on individual needs, individuals with Gastroparesis can navigate their dietary choices with confidence, ultimately fostering an improved quality of life. Remember, the goal is to create a sustainable and enjoyable eating plan that supports overall well-being while managing the challenges of Gastroparesis.

Complications If the Right Diet isn't Adopted.

When individuals with Gastroparesis do not adopt the right diet, they expose themselves to a range of potential complications that can significantly impact their health and well-being. Gastroparesis, characterized by delayed stomach emptying, requires careful dietary management to mitigate symptoms and prevent adverse outcomes. Here's an exploration of the complications that may arise when the right diet is not adopted:

1. Malnutrition: Gastroparesis can impede the proper absorption of essential nutrients, leading to malnutrition. Without adopting a diet tailored to the condition, individuals may not receive adequate vitamins, minerals, and calories, contributing to nutritional deficiencies.

2. Weight Loss: The delayed stomach emptying in Gastroparesis often results in reduced food intake. Without adhering to a proper diet, individuals may experience unintended weight loss, further compromising their nutritional status and overall health.

3. Dehydration: Gastroparesis can lead to decreased fluid intake due to symptoms like nausea and early satiety. Failing to adopt a diet that includes hydrating foods or fluids can result in dehydration, impacting various bodily functions and exacerbating symptoms.

4. Electrolyte Imbalance: Reduced food and fluid intake can disrupt electrolyte balance in the body. This imbalance, including deficiencies in sodium, potassium, and other electrolytes, can lead to complications such as muscle weakness, cramps, and irregular heart rhythms.

5. Gastrointestinal Obstruction (Bezoars): Gastroparesis increases the risk of bezoar formation, which are solid masses of undigested food that can accumulate in the stomach. Without a proper diet that facilitates digestion, bezoars can obstruct the gastrointestinal tract, causing severe pain, nausea, and vomiting.

6. Blood Sugar Fluctuations (for Diabetic Gastroparesis): Diabetic Gastroparesis, often associated with diabetes mellitus, can result in erratic blood sugar levels. Failing to adopt a suitable diet can exacerbate these fluctuations, making it challenging to manage diabetes effectively.

7. Worsening of Symptoms: Certain foods can exacerbate Gastroparesis symptoms, including nausea, vomiting, abdominal pain, and bloating. Without adopting a diet that considers individual triggers, these symptoms may intensify, significantly impacting the individual's quality of life.

8. Decreased Quality of Life: Persistent symptoms and complications resulting from an inadequate diet can significantly decrease the overall quality of life for individuals with Gastroparesis. Limited food choices, discomfort, and the impact on daily activities can lead to emotional distress and a diminished sense of well-being.

9. Increased Hospitalizations: Complications such as dehydration, malnutrition, and bezoar-related obstructions can necessitate hospitalization for individuals with Gastroparesis. Failing to adopt the right diet may increase the frequency and duration of hospital stays, disrupting normal daily life.

10. Medication Ineffectiveness:

Medications prescribed to manage Gastroparesis symptoms may be less effective without the support of a suitable diet. Inadequate nutrition and improper food choices can hinder the optimal functioning of medications, leading to suboptimal symptom relief.

Adopting the right diet is paramount for individuals with Gastroparesis to manage symptoms effectively and prevent potentially serious complications. Malnutrition, weight loss, dehydration, electrolyte imbalance, gastrointestinal obstructions, blood sugar fluctuations, worsening symptoms, decreased quality of life, and increased hospitalizations are all potential consequences of neglecting the dietary aspect of Gastroparesis management. It underscores the importance of working closely with healthcare professionals and registered dietitians to develop and adhere to a personalized Gastroparesis-friendly diet, allowing individuals to better navigate the challenges posed by this gastrointestinal disorder and optimize their overall health and well-being.

CHAPTER 3: MEAL PLANNING & PREPARATION

In the journey to manage gastroparesis, strategic meal planning and preparation become invaluable tools for individuals seeking a balance between nourishment and digestive comfort. This chapter serves as a guide, emphasizing the importance of thoughtful consideration when crafting meals.

Unlocking Culinary Success: Meal planning isn't just about ensuring a plate full of nutrients; it's a tailored approach to aligning individual tastes, preferences, and nutritional needs. Discover how to create a roadmap for your week, incorporating diverse flavors while adhering to the principles of a gastroparesis-friendly diet.

Efficiency in the Kitchen: From efficient grocery shopping to mastering batch cooking techniques, this section equips readers with practical skills to streamline the cooking process. Learn how to make the most of your time in the kitchen, minimizing stress and maximizing the enjoyment of nourishing, home-cooked meals.

Adaptability and Customization: Gastroparesis affects individuals differently, and this chapter emphasizes the flexibility required in meal planning. Explore ways to adapt recipes, swap ingredients, and personalize meals to suit your unique needs, ensuring a satisfying and manageable dining experience.

Embark on a culinary journey where planning and preparation become allies, empowering you to navigate the intricacies of gastroparesis with confidence and creativity.

Tips for Successful Gastroparesis Meal Planning

Meal planning for gastroparesis involves a thoughtful and strategic approach to ensure a balance between nutritional needs and digestive comfort. Here are essential tips to guide you towards successful meal planning tailored to the challenges of gastroparesis.

1. Know Your Triggers: Identify specific foods that trigger symptoms and customize your meal plan accordingly. Keep a food journal to track reactions and adjust your diet based on personal observations.

2. Prioritize Nutrient-Dense Foods: Opt for nutrient-dense options to ensure you receive essential vitamins and minerals. Focus on lean proteins, cooked vegetables, and easily digestible fruits to support your overall health.

3. Small, Frequent Meals: Break your daily intake into smaller, more frequent meals to reduce the strain on your digestive system. This approach helps manage symptoms by providing a steady supply of nutrients without overwhelming your stomach.

4. Hydrate Strategically: Stay hydrated, but be mindful of the timing. Consuming liquids with meals may lead to early satiety. Consider hydrating between meals to avoid diluting digestive juices during the critical phases of digestion.

5. Fiber Management: Opt for low-fiber choices to minimize digestive challenges. Cooked and peeled fruits and vegetables, white rice, and refined grains are gentler on the stomach compared to their high-fiber counterparts.

6. Balanced Plate Approach: Strive for a balanced plate that includes a combination of protein, carbohydrates, and healthy fats. This approach ensures a well-rounded mix of nutrients while considering the limitations of gastroparesis.

7. Mindful Cooking Techniques: Experiment with cooking techniques that enhance digestibility. Steaming, baking, and grilling can make food more palatable and easier to digest compared to frying or heavy sauces.

8. Create a Weekly Menu: Plan your meals for the week in advance, taking into account your schedule and energy levels. Having a structured menu reduces decision fatigue and allows you to prepare for the specific dietary needs associated with gastroparesis.

9. Batch Cooking and Freezing: Simplify meal preparation by batch cooking gastroparesis-friendly recipes. Divide portions into manageable servings and freeze them for quick and convenient meals, saving time and effort on busy days.

10. Supplement Wisely: Consult with your healthcare provider about necessary supplements to fill potential nutritional gaps. Vitamin and mineral supplements may be beneficial for gastroparesis patients, ensuring adequate nutrition despite dietary restrictions.

11. Listen to Your Body: Pay attention to your body's signals and adjust your meal plan accordingly. If certain

foods or portion sizes cause discomfort, be flexible and make necessary modifications to promote digestive ease.

12. Consult a Dietitian: Seek guidance from a registered dietitian experienced in managing gastroparesis. A professional can provide personalized advice, helping you create a meal plan that meets your nutritional needs while addressing the challenges posed by gastroparesis.

13. Embrace Variety: Keep your meals interesting by incorporating a variety of flavors, textures, and cooking styles. Experiment with herbs and spices to enhance taste without compromising on digestive comfort.

In conclusion, successful gastroparesis meal planning involves a combination of awareness, creativity, and adaptability. By understanding your body's responses, prioritizing nutrient-dense choices, and employing practical strategies, you can navigate the complexities of gastroparesis with confidence, ensuring a satisfying and nourishing culinary experience.

Batch Cooking and Freezing Techniques for Gastroparesis Meal Preparation

Efficient meal preparation is a cornerstone of managing gastroparesis, and batch cooking paired with freezing techniques can be transformative. These strategies not only save time and energy but also ensure a consistent supply of gastroparesis-friendly meals. Here's a comprehensive guide to mastering batch cooking and freezing for individuals navigating the challenges of gastroparesis.

1. Choose Freezer-Friendly Recipes: Opt for recipes that freeze well without compromising texture or flavor. Soups, stews, casseroles, and certain types of proteins like grilled chicken or turkey meatballs are excellent candidates for batch cooking and freezing.

2. Invest in Quality Containers: Use high-quality, airtight containers or freezer bags to store your meals. Proper packaging prevents freezer burn and maintains the integrity of the food. Consider portioning meals into single servings for convenient defrosting.

3. Label and Date: Clearly label each container with the name of the dish and the date it was prepared. This practice

helps you keep track of the contents in your freezer, ensuring you consume meals within a reasonable timeframe for optimal freshness.

4. Portion Control: Divide batch-cooked meals into individual portions to facilitate portion control. This approach not only simplifies meal planning but also allows you to thaw and heat only what you need, minimizing waste.

5. Cook Once, Eat Twice: Capitalize on cooking sessions by preparing double batches of gastroparesis-friendly recipes. Enjoy one portion immediately and freeze the second for later use. This method maximizes efficiency and extends the benefits of your culinary efforts.

6. Flash-Freezing Technique: For items like berries, diced fruits, or vegetables, employ the flash-freezing technique. Spread individual pieces on a baking sheet and freeze them before transferring to a container. This prevents the formation of clumps, allowing you to easily grab a handful for smoothies or quick snacks.

7. Consider Freeze-Friendly Ingredients: Some ingredients fare better in the freezer than others. Cooked grains, such as

rice or quinoa, and sauces can be frozen successfully. Avoid freezing items with high water content, like lettuce or cucumbers, as they may become mushy upon thawing.

8. Thawing Strategies: Plan ahead for mealtime by thawing frozen meals in the refrigerator overnight. This gradual thawing process helps maintain the texture and flavor of the food. Alternatively, use the defrost function on your microwave for quicker thawing.

9. Vacuum-Sealing Benefits: Consider investing in a vacuum sealer for added protection against freezer burn. Vacuum-sealed bags remove excess air, preserving the quality of the food for an extended period. This is particularly beneficial for longer-term storage.

10. Reheat with Care: When reheating frozen meals, use gentle methods such as stovetop simmering or microwave reheating to prevent overcooking. Add a splash of broth or water to maintain moisture levels, especially for dishes prone to drying out.

11. Rotate Stock Regularly: Keep track of your frozen inventory and practice the "first in, first out" approach.

Rotate older meals to the front of the freezer to ensure you consume them before introducing new additions.

12. Versatility in Ingredients: Choose versatile ingredients that can be incorporated into various dishes. For example, a batch of grilled chicken can be used in salads, wraps, or as a protein component in different main courses, providing variety without additional cooking efforts.

By integrating batch cooking and freezing techniques into your gastroparesis meal preparation routine, you gain a practical and time-saving approach to consistently enjoying nourishing meals. These strategies not only align with the dietary needs of gastroparesis but also empower individuals to navigate their culinary journey with ease and convenience.

Adapting Recipes to Personal Tastes and Needs for Gastroparesis

Navigating a gastroparesis-friendly diet doesn't mean sacrificing flavor or individual preferences. Adapting recipes to suit personal tastes and needs is a creative and empowering approach that allows individuals to enjoy satisfying meals while managing their condition. Here's a comprehensive guide on how to customize recipes for optimal taste and digestive comfort.

1. Ingredient Substitutions: Identify gastroparesis-friendly substitutes for ingredients that may trigger symptoms. For instance, replace high-fiber grains with lower-fiber alternatives like white rice or quinoa. Experiment with alternatives to find what works best for you.

2. Texture Modification: Gastroparesis often requires a focus on softer textures. Modify recipes by pureeing or mashing vegetables and fruits to achieve a smoother consistency. This technique not only enhances digestibility but also opens up opportunities for creative presentations.

3. Explore Herb and Spice Blends: Elevate the flavor profile of your dishes with herbs and spices. Experiment with blends that complement your palate without causing discomfort. Common choices include ginger, turmeric, basil, and mint, which add depth without overwhelming the digestive system.

4. Personalized Sauces and Broths: Craft personalized sauces and broths using gastroparesis-friendly ingredients. Create a light vegetable broth or a lemon-infused olive oil

drizzle to enhance the taste of your meals. These additions provide moisture and flavor without compromising digestive ease.

5. Customizable Proteins: Tailor protein sources to your liking. Whether it's choosing lean meats, poultry, fish, or plant-based proteins, select options that align with your taste preferences. Experiment with different cooking methods to find what suits your palate and digestive comfort.

6. Control Portion Sizes: Adjust portion sizes based on your individual tolerance levels. Smaller, more frequent meals can be easier to digest, preventing feelings of fullness and discomfort associated with larger servings.

7. Mindful Use of Fats: While gastroparesis-friendly recipes often limit fats, choose sources that agree with your system. Opt for heart-healthy fats found in avocados, olive oil, or nuts, and be mindful of portion sizes to avoid overwhelming your digestive capacity.

8. Experiment with Cooking Techniques: Explore cooking techniques that enhance flavor without compromising digestibility. Grilling, baking, and steaming are gentle

methods that retain the natural taste of ingredients while promoting easy digestion.

9. Build Flavor Gradually: Build layers of flavor gradually to create a well-balanced dish. Instead of relying on heavy seasonings, introduce flavors step by step, allowing your palate to appreciate the subtleties of each ingredient.

10. Create Custom Spice Blends: Develop your own spice blends tailored to your preferences and gastroparesis needs. Mixtures of cumin, coriander, and mild herbs can add depth to dishes without causing digestive distress.

11. Personalized Snack Choices: Adapt snacks to your liking by choosing easily digestible options. Customizable snacks include yogurt with low-fiber fruit, smooth nut butters, or small portions of crackers. Personalizing snacks allows for enjoyable nibbles throughout the day.

12. Intuitive Cooking: Embrace intuitive cooking by tasting and adjusting as you go. This approach allows you to tailor recipes in real-time, ensuring that the final dish aligns with your taste preferences and digestive requirements.

13. Consult with a Dietitian: Seek guidance from a registered dietitian specializing in gastroparesis. A professional can provide personalized advice based on your individual needs, helping you navigate recipe adaptations for optimal satisfaction and well-being.

Adapting recipes to personal tastes and needs is a dynamic and rewarding process. By experimenting with ingredients, textures, and flavors, individuals with gastroparesis can create a diverse and enjoyable menu that aligns with their unique preferences while supporting digestive comfort. This approach not only enhances the culinary experience but also contributes to the overall well-being of individuals managing gastroparesis.

Chapter 4: Dining Out and Social Situations

Navigating social occasions and dining out can be a nuanced challenge for individuals managing gastroparesis. Chapter 9 serves as a practical guide, offering insights and strategies to maintain both dietary adherence and social engagement. From choosing gastroparesis-friendly options on restaurant menus to effectively communicating dietary needs, this chapter empowers readers to navigate diverse social settings with confidence. Discover ways to strike a balance between enjoying shared meals and managing gastroparesis symptoms, ensuring that social interactions remain fulfilling and inclusive. With practical tips and mindful approaches, this chapter equips individuals to embrace the social aspect of dining while prioritizing their unique dietary requirements.

Strategies for Gastroparesis-Friendly Restaurant Choices

Dining out with gastroparesis requires a thoughtful approach to ensure an enjoyable experience without exacerbating symptoms. Implementing strategic strategies when choosing restaurants can make the difference between a satisfying meal and digestive discomfort. Here are practical tips to help you make gastroparesis-friendly restaurant choices:

1. Research Ahead: Prior to dining out, research restaurant menus online. Look for establishments that offer a variety of cooked, easily digestible options. Check for customizable choices or menu items that can be adapted to suit your specific dietary needs.

2. Choose Simple Preparations: Opt for dishes with straightforward preparations. Grilled, baked, or steamed options are often gentler on the digestive system compared to fried or heavily sauced dishes. Requesting minimal seasoning or sauces can further accommodate your needs.

3. Select Smaller Portions: Choose restaurants that offer smaller portion sizes or appetizer options. Smaller meals can be easier to manage, preventing feelings of fullness and discomfort associated with larger servings.

4. Embrace Flexibility: Be open to adapting menu items to suit your needs. Most restaurants are willing to accommodate dietary requests, such as omitting certain

ingredients or adjusting cooking methods. Don't hesitate to communicate your preferences to the server.

5. Prioritize Protein-Rich Options: Focus on protein-rich choices to support your nutritional needs. Grilled chicken, fish, or tofu are often well-tolerated and can be paired with cooked vegetables or easily digestible grains.

6. Inquire about Cooking Methods: Ask your server about the cooking methods used in specific dishes. Grilled or baked options are generally preferable to fried alternatives, as they are less likely to cause digestive distress.

7. Communicate Dietary Needs Clearly: Don't be afraid to communicate your dietary needs to the restaurant staff. Explain your condition, mentioning the importance of easily digestible, low-fiber options. Clear communication can lead to a more positive dining experience.

8. Plan Meal Timing: Consider planning your meal timing strategically. Choosing less busy times can result in more attentive service and may allow the kitchen to accommodate specific requests more effectively.

9. Explore Ethnic Cuisines: Explore ethnic cuisines known for their emphasis on simpler, well-cooked ingredients. Mediterranean, Japanese, or Mexican cuisines often offer diverse and gastroparesis-friendly options.

10. Beverage Choices Matter: Pay attention to beverage choices. Opt for still water, herbal teas, or clear broths to accompany your meal. Avoid carbonated and caffeinated beverages, as they can contribute to bloating and discomfort.

11. Bring Your Own Sauce: - Consider bringing your own gastroparesis-friendly sauce or dressing. This ensures you have a flavorful option that aligns with your dietary needs, even if the restaurant's offerings may not be suitable.

12. Scout Local Favorites: Ask locals or consult online reviews to discover gastroparesis-friendly restaurants in your area. Local favorites often prioritize fresh, simple ingredients, making them more conducive to managing digestive conditions.

13. Be Prepared with Snacks: Carry gastroparesis-friendly snacks in your bag. In case the restaurant options are

limited, having a small snack can help you maintain energy levels without compromising your dietary goals.

14. Create a List of Go-To Restaurants: Establish a list of go-to restaurants that consistently offer gastroparesis-friendly options. Having a reliable selection of eateries simplifies the decision-making process when dining out.

Navigating restaurants with gastroparesis demands a blend of proactiveness and flexibility. By researching, communicating effectively, and making informed choices, individuals can enjoy dining out without compromising their dietary goals. These strategies empower individuals to engage in social situations while prioritizing their unique needs and maintaining digestive well-being.

Communicating Dietary Needs to Others with Sensitivity and Clarity

Effectively communicating dietary needs, especially when managing conditions like gastroparesis, is essential for fostering understanding and support from friends, family, and those in social settings. Clear communication ensures that others can play a role in creating an environment that aligns with your specific dietary requirements. Here are key strategies to articulate your needs with sensitivity and clarity:

1. Educate and Advocate: Start by educating those around you about gastroparesis. Explain the condition, its impact on digestion, and the specific dietary considerations. This knowledge lays the foundation for understanding and empathy.

2. Choose the Right Moment: Timing is crucial when discussing dietary needs. Choose a calm, private moment to share information, ensuring that others can focus on your needs without distractions.

3. Be Direct and Specific: Clearly express your dietary restrictions and specific needs. Use straightforward language to communicate what you can and cannot consume. For example, mention the importance of low-fiber, easily digestible foods.

4. Share Personal Experiences: Personalize the conversation by sharing your experiences with gastroparesis. Discuss how certain foods impact your well-being and describe the symptoms you may experience if dietary needs are not met.

5. Provide Examples: Offer examples of foods that are suitable for your condition. This helps others understand the practical aspects of your dietary preferences and encourages them to make informed choices when planning meals or gatherings.

6. Offer Alternatives: Suggest alternative food options that align with your needs. This proactive approach makes it easier for others to accommodate your dietary requirements, especially in group settings or shared meals.

7. Utilize Positive Language: Frame your communication positively. Instead of focusing on restrictions, emphasize the variety of delicious and satisfying foods that are compatible with your dietary needs. This positive approach encourages cooperation and support.

8. Collaborate on Meal Planning: When participating in group meals, collaborate on meal planning. Work together to choose restaurants or prepare dishes that cater to your dietary needs while ensuring others can also enjoy the meal.

9. Offer to Contribute: Offer to contribute to meals or gatherings by preparing a dish that aligns with your dietary

requirements. This not only ensures you have a suitable option but also shows your commitment to participating in shared experiences.

10. Create a Dietary Card: Consider creating a small card summarizing your dietary needs. This card can be shared with hosts, chefs, or friends when planning meals, providing a quick reference for accommodating your requirements.

11. Express Gratitude: Acknowledge the efforts of those who support your dietary needs. Express gratitude for their understanding and willingness to make adjustments, fostering a positive and collaborative atmosphere.

12. Stay Open to Questions: Be open to questions and clarify any misconceptions. Encourage others to ask about your dietary needs, as this fosters a deeper understanding and helps dispel any uncertainties.

13. Address Social Situations Proactively: When attending social events, inform the host or organizer in advance about your dietary needs. This proactive communication allows for better planning and ensures that suitable options are available.

14. Share Resources: Share resources, such as articles or reputable websites, that provide additional information on gastroparesis and dietary recommendations. This can serve as a supplementary source for those who wish to learn more.

Effectively communicating dietary needs is a collaborative process that involves sharing information, offering alternatives, and fostering a supportive environment. By approaching these conversations with sensitivity, clarity, and a positive mindset, individuals with gastroparesis can build understanding and create a network of support that enhances their overall well-being.

Balancing Social Life with Nutritional Goals when Managing Gastroparesis

Maintaining a vibrant social life while managing gastroparesis requires a delicate balance between participating in gatherings and adhering to dietary restrictions. By adopting practical strategies, individuals can navigate social situations with confidence, ensuring a fulfilling and enjoyable experience while prioritizing their nutritional goals.

1. Open Communication: Communicate openly with friends and loved ones about your dietary needs. Sharing information about gastroparesis and explaining how certain foods impact your well-being helps set the stage for understanding and support.

2. Plan Ahead for Gatherings: Plan ahead when attending social events. If possible, inquire about the menu or suggest venues that offer gastroparesis-friendly options. This proactive approach ensures that you can participate in shared meals without compromising your nutritional goals.

3. Bring Your Own Dish: Consider bringing your own gastroparesis-friendly dish to gatherings. This not only guarantees a suitable option for you but also introduces others to delicious alternatives that align with your dietary needs.

4. Embrace Potluck Style Gatherings: Propose potluck-style gatherings where each attendee contributes a dish. This approach allows you to control the content of at least one dish, ensuring a safe and enjoyable option for yourself.

5. Focus on the Social Aspect: Shift the focus of social gatherings from food to shared experiences. Engage in

activities that don't revolve solely around meals, such as outdoor activities, game nights, or cultural events. This ensures that social connections remain strong without relying heavily on food-related interactions.

6. Educate Friends and Family: Educate your close circle about the impact of gastroparesis on your diet. Help them understand the importance of your nutritional goals and how they can play a supportive role in creating inclusive social environments.

7. Explore Gastroparesis-Friendly Restaurants: Explore and suggest restaurants known for their gastroparesis-friendly options. This proactive approach allows you to enjoy dining out while minimizing the stress associated with navigating unfamiliar menus.

8. Establish Regular Social Routines: Establish regular social routines that align with your dietary needs. Whether it's a weekly game night or a monthly gathering, creating predictable social events allows you to plan and prepare accordingly.

9. Create a Supportive Social Network: Surround yourself with a supportive social network that values your well-

being. Seek friends who understand your dietary restrictions and are willing to explore alternative ways of connecting that don't solely revolve around meals.

10. Develop Quick and Easy Recipes: Equip yourself with a repertoire of quick and easy gastroparesis-friendly recipes. Having simple go-to dishes allows you to prepare meals efficiently when socializing involves shared meals.

11. Choose Quality Over Quantity: Prioritize the quality of social interactions over the quantity of food consumed. Focus on the joy of connecting with others, and don't let dietary restrictions overshadow the richness of shared experiences.

12. Be Honest About Limitations: Be honest about your limitations when it comes to certain foods or meal settings. True friends will appreciate your honesty and support your efforts to maintain your nutritional goals.

13. Celebrate Achievements Together: Celebrate achievements together that don't involve food. Whether it's reaching personal goals, milestones, or shared successes, acknowledge and celebrate these moments without relying on traditional food-centric celebrations.

14. Offer Alternatives at Home: When hosting social events at home, offer a variety of gastroparesis-friendly alternatives. This ensures that your guests have options while allowing you to create an inclusive environment that aligns with your dietary needs.

Balancing social life with nutritional goals is a dynamic process that requires adaptability and creativity. By fostering understanding, planning ahead, and prioritizing social connections, individuals with gastroparesis can confidently engage in a fulfilling social life without compromising their dietary well-being.

Chapter 5: Beyond the Plate – Holistic Approaches

In the journey of managing gastroparesis, a holistic perspective extends beyond dietary choices. Chapter 10 delves into holistic approaches that encompass not only what's on the plate but also the broader aspects of well-being. From mindful eating practices to stress management techniques and the incorporation of exercise, this chapter explores how holistic strategies contribute to overall health. By embracing a comprehensive approach, individuals with gastroparesis can cultivate a balanced lifestyle that nurtures not only their physical health but also their mental and emotional well-being. Discover the interconnected nature of holistic approaches and how they synergize to enhance the quality of life for those navigating the complexities of gastroparesis.

Mindful Eating Practices for Managing Gastroparesis

Mindful eating is a powerful practice that can significantly impact the well-being of individuals managing gastroparesis. By fostering a heightened awareness of the eating experience, mindful eating not only enhances digestion but also cultivates a positive relationship with food. Here are key principles and practices for incorporating mindfulness into your eating routine:

1. Present-Moment Awareness: Engage in meals with full present-moment awareness. Be conscious of the sights, smells, and textures of your food. Minimize distractions such as phones or television to fully savor the eating experience.

2. Appreciation of Food: Cultivate gratitude for the nourishment your food provides. Acknowledge the effort that went into preparing the meal and express appreciation for the flavors and sustenance it offers.

3. Slow and Mindful Chewing: Chew your food slowly and mindfully. This practice not only aids digestion but also allows you to savor the taste of each bite. Pay attention to the textures and sensations as you chew.

4. Listening to Hunger Cues: Tune into your body's hunger cues. Eat when you're hungry, and pause when you're satisfied. Mindful eating encourages a deeper connection with your body's signals, helping you avoid overeating.

5. Portion Awareness: Be mindful of portion sizes. Use smaller plates and bowls to naturally control portions. This approach aligns with gastroparesis dietary guidelines, promoting smaller, more manageable meals.

6. Conscious Food Choices: Make conscious and intentional food choices. Consider the nutritional value and compatibility with your gastroparesis-friendly diet. Mindful eating encourages thoughtful decisions that support your overall health.

7. Mind-Body Connection: Foster a strong mind-body connection during meals. Listen to how your body responds to different foods and textures. This awareness can guide your dietary choices, minimizing discomfort associated with gastroparesis.

8. Eliminate Distractions: Create a calm and distraction-free eating environment. Turn off electronic devices, step away from work, and allow yourself dedicated time for meals. Minimizing distractions enhances your focus on the act of eating.

9. Non-Judgmental Observation: Approach your eating experiences with non-judgmental observation. Be curious

about your preferences, notice how different foods affect you, and refrain from self-criticism. This attitude promotes a positive relationship with food.

10. Mindful Drinking: Extend mindfulness to your beverage choices. Sip fluids slowly and pay attention to how your body responds. Opt for hydrating options that complement your gastroparesis-friendly diet.

11. Engage Your Senses: Engage multiple senses while eating. Appreciate the visual appeal of your plate, savor the aromas, and delight in the textures. This multisensory approach enhances the overall eating experience.

12. Gratitude Practices: Incorporate gratitude practices into your meals. Before eating, take a moment to express gratitude for the nourishment in front of you. This positive mindset contributes to a more mindful and fulfilling eating experience.

13. Mindful Snacking: Extend mindfulness to snacking occasions. Choose gastroparesis-friendly snacks mindfully, paying attention to hunger cues and selecting options that align with your nutritional goals.

14. Reflect on Fullness: Pause periodically during your meal to reflect on your level of fullness. This reflection allows you to gauge whether you've eaten enough or if you need to adjust portion sizes.

Cultivating mindful eating practices can profoundly impact the management of gastroparesis. By incorporating these principles into your daily routine, you not only enhance the digestion of your meals but also foster a deeper connection with your body and a more positive relationship with food. Mindful eating becomes a valuable ally in the holistic approach to well-being for individuals navigating the complexities of gastroparesis.

Stress Management for Gastroparesis: Nurturing Well-Being Amid Challenges

Stress can significantly impact the symptoms of gastroparesis, exacerbating digestive issues and diminishing overall well-being. Therefore, incorporating effective stress management strategies is crucial for individuals navigating this condition. Here are practical approaches to cultivate a sense of calm and promote emotional balance:

1. Mindfulness and Meditation: Engage in mindfulness practices and meditation to center your mind and alleviate stress. Mindful breathing exercises and guided meditations can be particularly beneficial in fostering a sense of calm amidst the challenges of gastroparesis.

2. Deep Breathing Techniques: Practice deep breathing techniques to activate the body's relaxation response. Slow, intentional breaths can reduce stress hormones and promote a sense of tranquility, positively impacting both mental and physical well-being.

3. Gentle Exercise: Incorporate gentle exercise into your routine. Activities like walking, yoga, or tai chi not only contribute to physical health but also serve as effective stress-relieving practices. Consult with your healthcare provider to identify suitable exercise options.

4. Progressive Muscle Relaxation: Explore progressive muscle relaxation, a technique involving the gradual tensing and releasing of muscle groups. This approach helps release physical tension and promotes a state of relaxation.

5. Establish a Relaxing Routine: Establish a soothing routine before bedtime. Engage in activities that promote relaxation, such as reading, gentle stretching, or taking a warm bath. Quality sleep contributes significantly to stress management.

6. Cognitive-Behavioral Therapy (CBT): Consider cognitive-behavioral therapy (CBT) to address stress-related thoughts and behaviors. Working with a mental health professional trained in CBT can provide valuable tools for managing stress and improving overall well-being.

7. Journaling: Maintain a stress journal to identify triggers and patterns. Regularly jotting down your thoughts and emotions can offer insights into stressors specific to your situation, empowering you to address them effectively.

8. Seek Social Support: Foster social connections and seek support from friends, family, or support groups. Sharing your experiences and feelings can alleviate emotional burdens and provide a sense of community, contributing to stress reduction.

9. Set Realistic Goals: Establish realistic goals and expectations for yourself. Acknowledge the challenges

posed by gastroparesis and set achievable objectives. Breaking down larger tasks into smaller, manageable steps can alleviate stress associated with feeling overwhelmed.

10. Time Management: Prioritize time management to reduce stress associated with deadlines and commitments. Organize your schedule, set realistic timelines, and allocate breaks to prevent feelings of pressure and urgency.

11. Limit Stimulants: Minimize the consumption of stimulants like caffeine and nicotine, as they can contribute to increased stress levels. Choose hydrating and calming beverages, such as herbal teas or infused water.

12. Practice Gratitude: Cultivate a practice of gratitude. Regularly acknowledging and appreciating positive aspects of your life can shift focus away from stressors, fostering a more optimistic mindset.

13. Biofeedback Techniques: Explore biofeedback techniques with the guidance of a healthcare professional. Biofeedback allows you to gain awareness and control over physiological responses to stress, promoting relaxation and stress reduction.

14. Learn to Say No: Develop the ability to say no when necessary. Setting boundaries and recognizing your limitations are crucial for preventing overwhelm and minimizing stress associated with excessive commitments.

Effectively managing stress is an integral part of a holistic approach to gastroparesis care. By incorporating these strategies into your daily life, you can cultivate emotional resilience and create a supportive environment for your overall well-being. It's essential to recognize that stress management is a personal journey, and finding approaches that resonate with you is key to navigating the challenges of gastroparesis with grace and resilience.

Incorporating Exercise for Overall Well-being in Gastroparesis Management

Exercise plays a pivotal role in promoting overall well-being, especially for individuals managing conditions like gastroparesis. While it's important to tailor exercise routines to individual needs and limitations, incorporating physical activity can contribute significantly to both physical and mental health. Here are guidelines and considerations for integrating exercise into your gastroparesis management plan:

1. Consult with Healthcare Providers: Before starting any exercise regimen, consult with your healthcare provider, particularly if you have underlying health conditions. They can provide guidance on suitable exercises based on your specific health status and the severity of gastroparesis symptoms.

2. Choose Gentle Forms of Exercise: Opt for gentle forms of exercise that align with your comfort level and physical capabilities. Walking, swimming, and tai chi are low-impact options that can be adapted to accommodate varying energy levels and sensitivities.

3. Set Realistic Goals: Establish realistic and achievable exercise goals. Start with short durations and gradually increase intensity as your stamina improves. Consistency is key, and setting attainable goals ensures a sustainable and positive exercise experience.

4. Focus on Flexibility and Strength: Emphasize flexibility and strength training in your exercise routine. These components not only contribute to overall fitness but also

support joint mobility and muscle tone. Yoga and gentle strength exercises can be beneficial.

5. Prioritize Regular Movement: Prioritize regular movement throughout the day. Break up periods of sedentary behavior by incorporating short walks, stretches, or light exercises. Consistent, gentle movement can enhance circulation and alleviate feelings of stiffness.

6. Mindful Exercise Practices: Adopt mindful exercise practices that emphasize the mind-body connection. Engage in activities like yoga or tai chi that promote relaxation, stress reduction, and an awareness of your body's responses.

7. Modify Intensity Based on Symptoms: Be attentive to your body's signals and modify exercise intensity based on symptoms. If you experience fatigue or discomfort, consider gentler activities or reduce the duration of your exercise sessions. Listening to your body is crucial in managing gastroparesis.

8. Stay Hydrated: Maintain proper hydration, especially during exercise. Dehydration can exacerbate symptoms

associated with gastroparesis, so ensure you drink water before, during, and after your exercise sessions.

9. Consider Post-Meal Walks: Incorporate short walks after meals. Gentle post-meal walks can aid digestion and alleviate symptoms such as bloating. Aim for a leisurely stroll to avoid putting excessive stress on your digestive system.

10. Seek Professional Guidance: Consider seeking guidance from a fitness professional experienced in working with individuals managing health conditions. They can create personalized exercise plans that cater to your specific needs, taking gastroparesis symptoms into account.

11. Embrace Adaptability:

- Embrace adaptability in your exercise routine. Some days you may feel more energetic than others, and that's perfectly normal. Modify your exercise activities based on how you feel, allowing for flexibility and self-compassion.

12. Choose Enjoyable Activities: Select activities that you genuinely enjoy. Whether it's dancing, gardening, or gentle cycling, engaging in activities you find enjoyable increases

motivation and contributes to a positive exercise experience.

13. Monitor Stress Levels: Be mindful of stress levels and use exercise as a tool for stress management. Activities like deep breathing exercises or gentle yoga can help regulate stress hormones, fostering emotional well-being.

14. Track Progress and Adjust: Keep track of your exercise progress and adjust your routine as needed. Regularly reassess your goals and modify your exercise plan based on improvements, challenges, and feedback from your healthcare team.

Incorporating exercise into your gastroparesis management plan requires a thoughtful and individualized approach. By focusing on gentle, enjoyable activities and being mindful of your body's responses, you can enhance your overall well-being and contribute to the holistic care of gastroparesis. Always prioritize your health and consult with healthcare professionals to ensure that your exercise routine aligns with your specific needs and goals.

CHAPTER 6: GASTROPARESIS RECIPES

BREAKFAST RECIPES

Here are 10 Gastroparesis-friendly breakfast recipes designed to be gentle on the digestive system while providing essential nutrients. These recipes focus on easily digestible ingredients and preparation methods:

1. Banana and Almond Butter Smoothie:

Ingredients:

- 1 ripe banana
- 1 tablespoon almond butter (smooth)
- 1 cup almond milk (unsweetened)

Preparation:

1. In a blender, combine the ripe banana, almond butter, and almond milk.
2. Blend until smooth and creamy.
3. Pour into a glass and enjoy this nutrient-rich smoothie.

2. Oatmeal with Mashed Berries:

Ingredients:

- 1/2 cup rolled oats
- 1/2 cup mashed berries (blueberries, raspberries, or strawberries)
- 1 tablespoon honey (optional)

Preparation:

1. Cook the rolled oats according to package instructions.
2. Once cooked, stir in the mashed berries and honey.
3. Serve warm, providing a comforting and nutritious breakfast.

3. Greek Yogurt Parfait:

Ingredients:

- 1/2 cup Greek yogurt (low-fat)
- 1/4 cup granola (low-fat, low-fiber)
- 1/4 cup diced ripe mango

Preparation:

- In a glass or bowl, layer Greek yogurt, granola, and diced mango.
- Repeat the layers, creating a delicious and visually appealing parfait.

4. Scrambled Eggs with Spinach:

Ingredients:

- 2 eggs (beaten)
- 1/2 cup fresh spinach (chopped)
- Salt and pepper to taste

Preparation:

- In a non-stick pan, lightly sauté the chopped spinach until wilted.
- Pour in the beaten eggs, stirring gently until scrambled.
- Season with salt and pepper and serve, providing a protein-packed breakfast.

5. Mango Smoothie Bowl:

Ingredients:

- 1 cup frozen mango chunks

- 1/2 cup coconut milk (unsweetened)
- Toppings: sliced bananas, chia seeds, and shredded coconut

Preparation:

- Blend the frozen mango chunks with coconut milk until smooth.
- Pour the smoothie into a bowl and top with sliced bananas, chia seeds, and shredded coconut.

6. Rice Pudding with Cinnamon:

Ingredients:

- 1/2 cup cooked white rice
- 1/2 cup almond milk (unsweetened)
- 1 tablespoon honey
- Cinnamon for sprinkling

Preparation:

1. Mix the cooked white rice with almond milk and honey.
2. Sprinkle with cinnamon and warm in the microwave.

3. Enjoy a comforting rice pudding for breakfast.

7. Apple and Peanut Butter Wrap:

Ingredients:

- 1 whole-grain tortilla (soft)
- 1 tablespoon peanut butter (smooth)
- 1/2 apple (thinly sliced)

Preparation:

1. Spread peanut butter evenly on the tortilla.
2. Place sliced apples on one half of the tortilla, fold, and enjoy a quick and satisfying wrap.

8. Quinoa Porridge with Maple Syrup:

Ingredients:

- 1/2 cup cooked quinoa
- 1/2 cup almond milk (unsweetened)
- 1 tablespoon maple syrup
- Chopped nuts for garnish

Preparation:

1. Combine cooked quinoa, almond milk, and maple syrup.
2. Heat until warm and top with chopped nuts for added texture.

9. Cottage Cheese and Pineapple Bowl:

Ingredients:

- 1/2 cup cottage cheese
- 1/2 cup diced fresh pineapple
- 1 tablespoon sunflower seeds

Preparation:

1. Mix cottage cheese with diced pineapple.
2. Sprinkle sunflower seeds on top for a protein-packed, tropical breakfast bowl.

10. Blueberry Chia Seed Pudding:

Ingredients:

- 1/4 cup chia seeds
- 1 cup almond milk (unsweetened)
- 1/2 cup blueberries (fresh or frozen)

- Preparation:

1. Mix chia seeds and almond milk in a jar and refrigerate overnight.

2. In the morning, layer chia pudding with blueberries for a delightful and nutritious pudding.

These Gastroparesis diet breakfast recipes offer a variety of flavors and textures while prioritizing easy digestion and symptom management. Adjust portions and ingredients based on individual tolerances and preferences. Always consult with healthcare professionals or a registered dietitian for personalized advice.

LUNCH RECIPES

Here are 10 Gastroparesis-friendly lunch recipes designed to be gentle on the digestive system while providing essential nutrients. These recipes focus on easily digestible ingredients and preparation methods:

1. Chicken and Rice Soup:

Ingredients:

- 1 cup shredded cooked chicken
- 1/2 cup cooked white rice
- 1 cup chicken broth (low-fat, low-sodium)

Preparation:

1. Combine shredded chicken, cooked rice, and chicken broth in a pot.
2. Heat until warm and enjoy a comforting chicken and rice soup.

2. Salmon Salad with Avocado:

Ingredients:

- 1/2 cup canned salmon (drained)
- 1/2 avocado (diced)
- Mixed greens (lettuce, spinach)

Preparation:

1. Mix canned salmon with diced avocado.
2. Serve over a bed of mixed greens for a light and nutritious salmon salad.

3. Quinoa and Vegetable Stir-Fry:

Ingredients:

- 1/2 cup cooked quinoa
- Assorted vegetables (bell peppers, zucchini, carrots)
- 1 tablespoon olive oil

Preparation:

1. Sauté assorted vegetables in olive oil until tender.
2. Mix in cooked quinoa and stir-fry for a simple and flavorful lunch option.

4. Turkey and Mashed Sweet Potatoes:

Ingredients:

- 1/2 cup ground turkey (cooked)
- 1/2 cup mashed sweet potatoes
- Steamed green beans

Preparation:

1. Cook ground turkey until fully cooked.
2. Serve over mashed sweet potatoes with steamed green beans on the side.

5. Spinach and Feta Omelette:

Ingredients:

- 2 eggs (beaten)
- Handful of fresh spinach (chopped)
- 1 tablespoon feta cheese (crumbled)

Preparation:

1. Sauté chopped spinach until wilted.
2. Pour beaten eggs over the spinach, sprinkle with feta, and cook to make a delicious omelette.

6. Hummus and Turkey Wrap:

Ingredients:

- 1 whole-grain tortilla (soft)
- 2 tablespoons hummus
- 3 slices turkey (low-fat)

Preparation:

1. Spread hummus on the tortilla.
2. Place turkey slices on top, wrap, and enjoy a quick and satisfying lunch.

7. Miso Soup with Tofu and Bok Choy:

Ingredients:

- 1 cup miso soup (low-sodium)
- 1/2 cup tofu cubes
- Handful of bok choy (chopped)

Preparation:

1. Heat miso soup and add tofu cubes and chopped bok choy.
2. Simmer until tofu is heated through, creating a light and nourishing soup.

8. Baked Cod with Lemon and Dill:

Ingredients:

1. 1 piece cod fillet
2. 1 tablespoon olive oil
3. Fresh lemon slices and dill for garnish

Preparation:

1. Place cod fillet on a baking sheet, drizzle with olive oil, and add lemon slices and dill.
2. Bake until the fish is cooked through, providing a simple and flavorful main course.

9. Cottage Cheese and Pineapple Stuffed Bell Peppers:

Ingredients:

1. 1/2 cup cottage cheese

2.   1/2 cup diced fresh pineapple

3.   Mini bell peppers (halved and deseeded)

Preparation:

1.   Mix cottage cheese with diced pineapple.

2.   Stuff mini bell peppers with the cottage cheese and pineapple mixture for a refreshing lunch option.

10. Sweet Potato and Turkey Hash:

- Ingredients:

-   1/2 cup ground turkey (cooked)
-   1/2 cup sweet potatoes (diced and cooked)
-   Spinach leaves for garnish

- Preparation:

1.   Cook ground turkey until fully cooked.

2.   Combine with diced and cooked sweet potatoes, garnish with spinach leaves, and enjoy a hearty and nutritious hash.

These Gastroparesis diet lunch recipes offer a variety of flavors and textures while prioritizing easy digestion and symptom management. Adjust portions and ingredients based on individual tolerances and preferences. Always consult with healthcare professionals or a registered dietitian for personalized advice.

DINNER RECIPES

Here are 10 Gastroparesis-friendly dinner recipes designed to be gentle on the digestive system while providing essential nutrients. These recipes focus on easily digestible ingredients and preparation methods:

1. Baked Chicken and Mashed Potatoes:

Ingredients:

- 1 boneless, skinless chicken breast
- 1/2 cup mashed potatoes
- Steamed carrots for garnish

Preparation:

1. Season the chicken breast and bake until fully cooked.
2. Serve with a side of mashed potatoes and steamed carrots for a comforting and easy-to-digest dinner.

2. Shrimp and Quinoa Salad:

Ingredients:

1. 1/2 cup cooked shrimp

2. 1/2 cup cooked quinoa

3. Mixed greens (lettuce, spinach)

Preparation:

1. Combine cooked shrimp and quinoa.

2. Serve over a bed of mixed greens for a light and protein-packed salad.

3. Vegetarian Stir-Fry with Tofu:

Ingredients:

- 1/2 cup tofu cubes

- Assorted vegetables (broccoli, bell peppers, snap peas)

- 1 tablespoon soy sauce (low-sodium)

Preparation:

1. Sauté tofu cubes and assorted vegetables in a pan with low-sodium soy sauce.

2. Serve over white rice for a flavorful and easily digestible stir-fry.

4. Turkey and Rice Congee:

Ingredients:

- 1/2 cup ground turkey (cooked)
- 1/2 cup cooked white rice
- Chicken broth (low-fat, low-sodium)

Preparation:

1. Cook ground turkey until fully cooked.
2. Mix with cooked white rice and thin with low-fat, low-sodium chicken broth to make a comforting congee.

5. Salmon and Sweet Potato Mash:

Ingredients:

- 1 piece salmon fillet
- 1/2 cup mashed sweet potatoes
- Steamed green beans for garnish

Preparation:

1. Bake salmon until fully cooked.
2. Serve with a side of mashed sweet potatoes and steamed green beans for a nutritious dinner.

6. Egg Drop Soup with Spinach:

Ingredients:

- 2 eggs (beaten)
- 1 cup chicken broth (low-fat, low-sodium)
- Handful of fresh spinach (chopped)

Preparation:

1. Heat chicken broth and add beaten eggs, stirring gently.
2. Add chopped spinach and simmer until the eggs are cooked, creating a simple and nourishing egg drop soup.

7. Ground Chicken and Butternut Squash Skillet:

Ingredients:

- 1/2 cup ground chicken (cooked)
- 1/2 cup butternut squash (diced and cooked)
- Fresh herbs for garnish

Preparation:

1. Cook ground chicken until fully cooked.

2. Mix with diced and cooked butternut squash, garnish with fresh herbs, and enjoy a flavorful skillet dinner.

8. Lemon Herb Baked Cod:

Ingredients:

- 1 piece cod fillet
- Lemon juice, olive oil, fresh herbs (rosemary, thyme)

Preparation:

1. Drizzle cod fillet with lemon juice and olive oil, sprinkle with fresh herbs.
2. Bake until the fish is fully cooked, creating a light and aromatic baked cod.

9. Mashed Cauliflower and Turkey Patties:

Ingredients:

- 1/2 cup ground turkey (cooked)
- 1/2 cup mashed cauliflower
- Steamed asparagus for garnish

Preparation:

1. Cook ground turkey until fully cooked.

2. Serve with a side of mashed cauliflower and steamed asparagus for a low-carb and easily digestible dinner.

10. Pumpkin Soup with Chicken:

- Ingredients:

- 1 cup pumpkin puree
- Shredded cooked chicken
- Chicken broth (low-fat, low-sodium)

- Preparation:

1. Combine pumpkin puree, shredded cooked chicken, and low-fat, low-sodium chicken broth.
2. Heat until warm, creating a velvety pumpkin soup with protein.

These Gastroparesis diet dinner recipes offer a variety of flavors and textures while prioritizing easy digestion and symptom management. Adjust portions and ingredients based on individual tolerances and preferences. Always consult with healthcare professionals or a registered dietitian for personalized advice.

CONCLUSION

In conclusion, embracing a Gastroparesis diet is not merely a culinary adjustment; it is a proactive step towards reclaiming control over one's digestive health and overall well-being. This carefully curated approach to nutrition, tailored to accommodate the challenges posed by delayed stomach emptying, offers a spectrum of benefits. From symptom management and improved nutrient absorption to stabilized blood sugar levels (especially for those with diabetic Gastroparesis), the Gastroparesis diet plays a pivotal role in mitigating complications and enhancing the overall quality of life.

By prioritizing easily digestible foods, avoiding triggers, and maintaining a balanced approach to nutrition, individuals with Gastroparesis can experience relief from symptoms, prevent nutritional deficiencies, and foster a sense of empowerment in managing their health. The recipes provided, spanning breakfast, lunch, and dinner options, underscore the versatility and richness of a Gastroparesis-friendly diet, demonstrating that dietary restrictions need not equate to culinary monotony.

As you embark on this journey, remember that adopting and adapting to a Gastroparesis diet is not just a dietary shift; it is a commitment to self-care and resilience. Each meal becomes a nourishing opportunity to support your body, alleviate discomfort, and cultivate a positive relationship with food. Motivation arises from the prospect of regaining control over your health narrative, savoring flavorful, gentle-on-the-stomach meals, and ultimately enjoying an improved quality of life. Your journey to wellness starts with the choices you make daily—choices that prioritize your health, well-being, and a future filled with vitality. Embrace the Gastroparesis diet not as a constraint, but as a gateway to a more vibrant and fulfilling life. Your body deserves the nourishment that empowers it to thrive, and your journey towards optimal health begins with the mindful choices you make in every meal.

CONTACT US

FREE 30 DAYS MEAL PLANNER

FREE 30Days Meal Planner, a priceless extra to get you started on the path to a more organized and healthy living. This meticulously curated planner is made to make meal planning easier, save you time, and help you meet your nutritional objectives. Prepare to enjoy the advantages of this wonderful resource! Scan the QR Code below now.

www.ingramcontent.com/pod-product-compliance
Lightning Source LLC
Chambersburg PA
CBHW060946260726
48661CB00005B/1784